AT HOME IN YOUR BODY

CARE FOR THE SHAPE YOU'RE IN

OBESITY & KIDS

BIGGER ISN'T ALWAYS BETTER:
CHOOSING YOUR PORTIONS

COOKIES OR CARROTS? YOU ARE WHAT YOU EAT

WEIGHTED DOWN:
WHEN BEING OVERWEIGHT MAKES YOU SICK

GETTING STRONGER, GETTING FIT:
THE IMPORTANCE OF EXERCISE

THE TRUTH ABOUT DIETS:
WHAT'S RIGHT FOR YOU?

TIRED OF BEING TEASED:
OBESITY AND OTHERS

DOES TELEVISION MAKE YOU FAT?
LIFESTYLE AND OBESITY

TOO MANY SUNDAY DINNERS:
FAMILY AND DIET

I EAT WHEN I'M SAD:
FOOD AND FEELINGS

AT HOME IN YOUR BODY:
CARE FOR THE SHAPE YOU'RE IN

AT HOME IN YOUR BODY

CARE FOR THE SHAPE YOU'RE IN

BY RAE SIMONS

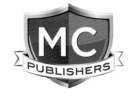

MC
PUBLISHERS

Mason Crest Publishers

MASON CREST PUBLISHERS INC.
370 Reed Road
Broomall, Pennsylvania 19008
(866)MCP-BOOK (toll free)
www.masoncrest.com

First Printing
9 8 7 6 5 4 3 2 1

Library of Congress Cataloging-in-Publication Data

Simons, Rae, 1957–
  At home in your body : care for the shape you're in / by Rae Simons.
      p. cm. — (Obesity & kids)
  Includes bibliographical references and index.
    ISBN 978-1-4222-1715-3 (hardcover)   ISBN 978-1-4222-1705-4 (series)
    ISBN 978-1-4222-1903-4 (pbk.)   ISBN 978-1-4222-1893-8 (pbk. series)
  1. Self-care, Health. 2. Beauty, Personal. 3. Self-confidence in children. 4. Obesity in children. I. Title.
  RA776.95.S585 2010
  613—dc22
                        2010015436

Design by Wendy Arakawa.
Produced by Harding House Publishing Service, Inc.
www.hardinghousepages.com
Cover design by Torque Advertising and Design.
Printed in USA by Bang Printing.

CONTENTS

INTRODUCTION
FOR THE TEACHERS

We as a society often reserve our harshest criticism for those conditions we understand the least. Such is the case for obesity. Obesity is a chronic and often-fatal disease that accounts for 400,000 deaths each year. It is second only to smoking as a cause of premature death in the United States. People suffering from obesity need understanding, support, and medical assistance. Yet what they often receive is scorn.

Today, children are the fastest growing segment of the obese population in the United States. This constitutes a public health crisis of enormous proportions. Living with childhood obesity affects self-esteem, which down the road can affect employment and attainment of higher education. But childhood obesity is much more than a social stigma. It has serious health consequences.

Childhood obesity increases the risk for poor health in adulthood—but also even during childhood. Depression, diabetes, asthma, gallstones, orthopedic diseases, and other obesity-related conditions are all on the rise in children. Recent estimates suggest that 30 to 50 percent of children born in 2000 will develop type 2 diabetes mellitus, a leading cause of preventable blindness, kidney failure, heart disease, stroke, and amputations. Obesity is undoubtedly the most pressing nutritional disorder among young people today.

If we are to reverse obesity's current trend, there must be family, community, and national objectives promoting healthy eating and exercise. As a nation, we must demand broad-based public-health initiatives to limit TV watching, curtail junk food advertising toward children, and promote physical activity. More than rhetoric, these need to be our rallying cry. Anything short of this will eventually fail, and within our lifetime obesity will become the leading cause of death in the United States if not in the world. This series is an excellent first step in battling the obesity crisis by educating young children about the risks, the realities, and what they can do to build healthy lifestyles right now.

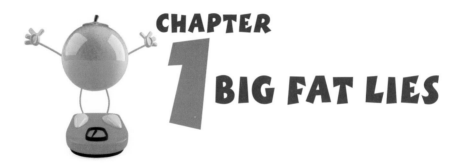

CHAPTER 1
BIG FAT LIES

Have you ever looked in the mirror and thought:

If only my hair were different?
If only my nose were a different shape?
If only I were skinnier?

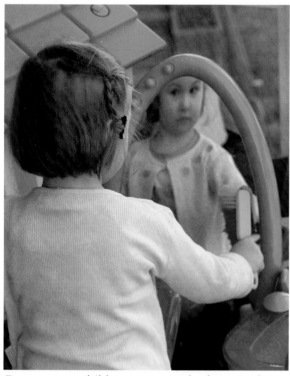

Even young children may not be happy about what they see when they look in the mirror.

Most people have thoughts like this sometimes. We feel as though people would like us more if we looked different. We even feel as though we'd be somehow worth more if we looked different. And we would definitely like ourselves better if we looked differ-ent! We don't feel at home in our own bodies.

But when we can't accept the way we look—when we don't even like ourselves because of the way we look—that's a problem.

AMAZING YOU

You are amazing and wonderful, no matter what you look like. Your brain works faster and better than any computer. Your eyes and ears take in light and vibrations, and then send messages to your brain, allowing you to see and hear. Your heart beats over and over and over, never resting for seventy, eighty, even one hundred years, sending blood through your veins every second of every day. Every moment, your body does all the complicated jobs that not only keep you alive but that also allow you to think, feel, talk, learn, play, laugh, cry, dream, and work. If you stop to really think about

DID YOU KNOW?

A stereotype is a picture we have in our heads about a group of people. It's not necessarily true. In fact, it seldom is, because people are individuals, and each person within a group is different. But many people have a stereotype in their heads when they think about people who are overweight and obese. Thinking of people who are overweight as "pigs" is just part of that stereotype—but pigs are also the victims of untrue stereotypes. In reality, pigs are not normally fat. If they have their choice, they are not normally dirty. And pigs are very intelligent. So remember: stereotypes are often simply not true!

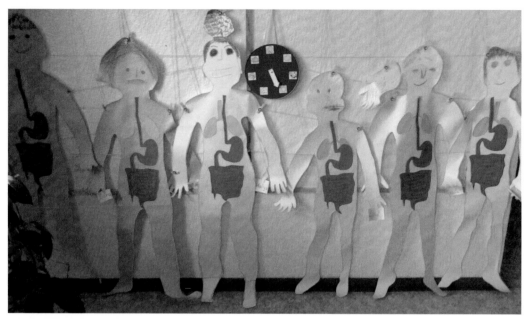

Every now and then, stop and think about all the amazing things your body lets you do!

it, you'll realize your body is a miracle. It takes in food and turns it into energy. It breathes in oxygen and sends it out to each of the tiny cells in your body. It's more magic than any wizard's spell!

BEING "PERFECT"

But many people in the world still don't like the way they look. They don't realize how wonderful their own bodies are. They criticize other people's bodies. They don't give their own bodies the love and respect they deserve. Instead, they hate their bodies—or they're not kind to others whose bodies don't measure up to the "perfect" **standard**. They make judgments about how nice or smart or interesting other people are based on what they look like. And they turn this same mean attitude against themselves.

So where did that "perfect" standard come from? Where do so many people get the idea that we should all look a certain way?

MEDIA MESSAGES

One of the big reasons so many people don't like the way they look is that they're picking up messages from the **media**—magazines, television, movies, and the Internet.

Think about the last movie you saw in a theater. What kind of people played the "good" guys, the people you liked? Were any of them fat, covered with pimples, or "ugly" in some way? Did any of them have bad hair, terrible makeup, funny-looking teeth, or ugly clothes? Now think about your favorite

What's a standard? It's something people use as the basis for comparison for everything else.

What's the media? The media is the various means of communication that reach large numbers of people.

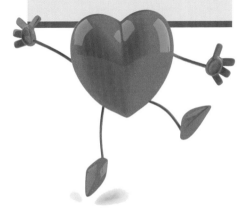

television shows, commercials, and music stars. How many of these stars are less-than-perfect people?

Probably not too many. But how about the bad guys? How do they dress? What do they look like? What about the scary people in a movie? Don't they often look "weird" in some way?

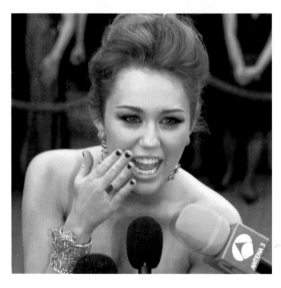

Stars like Miley Cyrus are beautiful, talented and seem to have perfect lives. Young fans often think they would be happier if they could be more like the stars they see on television and in movies.

They fall way short of that "perfect" standard we talked about earlier.

There's a message behind all this:

Good guys are beautiful. Bad guys are not.

Talented people, the people we admire and imitate, are good-looking and thin. People who have little to offer the world are funny looking and overweight. Important people are tan and

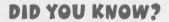

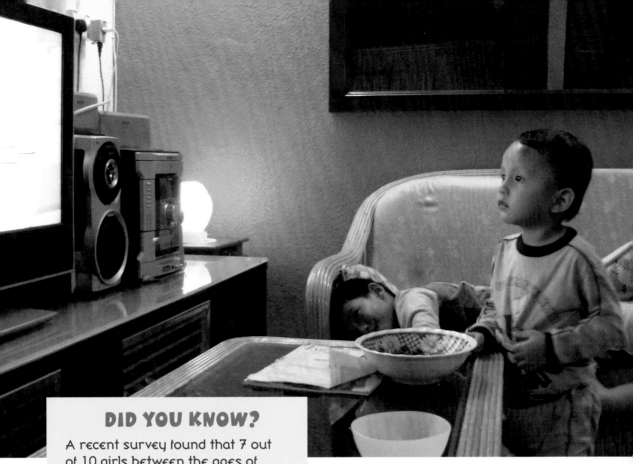

DID YOU KNOW?

A recent survey found that 7 out of 10 girls between the ages of 10 and 17 said they wanted to look like a television character. Nearly one-third said that they had changed their appearance to become more like a TV character. Sixteen percent (nearly 1 out of every 5) said that they had dieted or exercised to look more like a TV character.

According to the University of Michigan, on average children ages 2–5 spend 32 hours a week in front of a TV—watching television, DVDs, DVR and videos, and using a game console. Kids ages 6–11 spend about 28 hours a week in front of the TV.

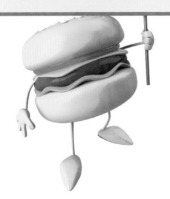

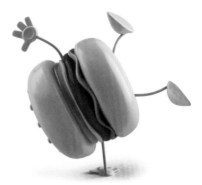

athletic and wear nice clothes. Worthless people are fat and wear ugly clothes.

Over and over, everywhere we turn, every day, in ads and commercials and television shows and movie videos, we see gorgeous models and actors who never have an ounce of fat on their bodies. Even little children can't help but pick up the message that if they want to be pretty or good-looking, they need to all look pretty much exactly the same way.

But this message is a big fat lie.

THE TRUTH

Here's what's the truth:

Everyone looks different—and that's okay.

Bodies come in lots of shapes and sizes—and that's okay.

There are many different kinds of pretty, and many different ways to be good-looking.

Being healthy is a lot more important than being perfect!

DID YOU KNOW?

We often think of pigs and fatness together. But pigs are also the victims of untrue stereotypes. In reality, pigs are not normally fat. If they have their choice, they are not normally dirty (they do like to roll in mud on hot, sunny days, but that's only because they get sunburned easily). And pigs are very intelligent. So remember: stereotypes are often simply not true! And that's not true.

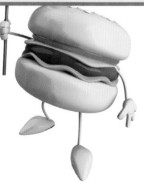

Every body is different. Learn what is healthiest for your own body—don't try to be like someone else.

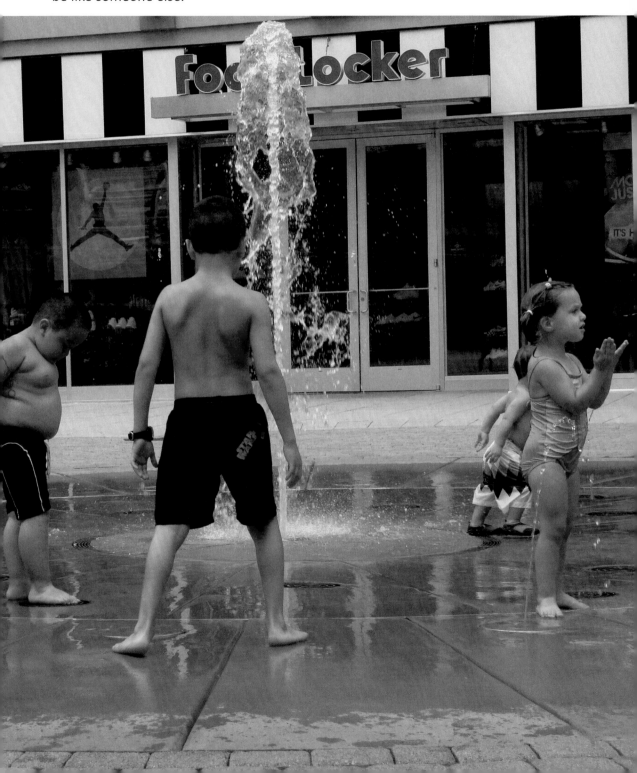

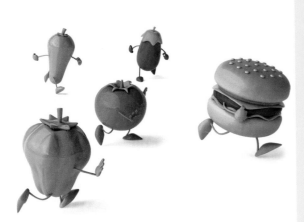

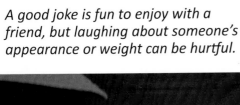

DID YOU KNOW?

Prejudice is the word we use when we think differently about others because of their race, their religion, or the way they look. Most of us know this is wrong—but many people think it's okay to think about people differently because they are overweight. This is a form of prejudice too. And yet we hear fat jokes at school all the time. Grownups tell fat jokes too. People on television do as well. Most of the time, people forget how cruel this is, or how it makes others feel.

A good joke is fun to enjoy with a friend, but laughing about someone's appearance or weight can be hurtful.

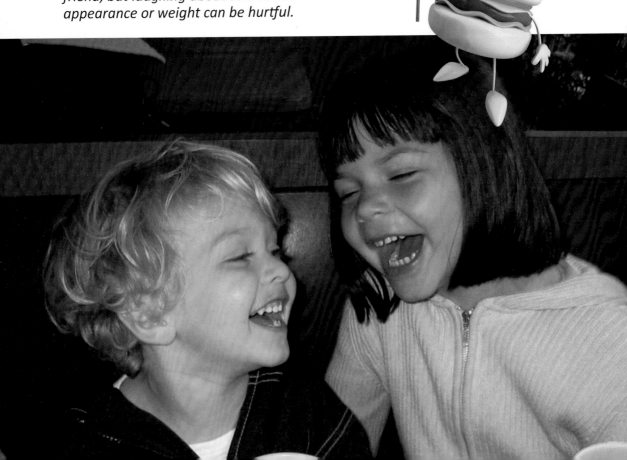

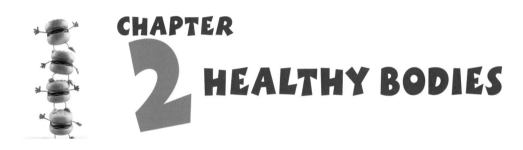

CHAPTER 2 HEALTHY BODIES

People have different ideas about what's beautiful. And over the years, their ideas often change. But good health doesn't change.

Look at pictures of your mom and dad when they were young. Chances are the clothes they were wearing and their hairstyles are pretty different from what people are wearing today. Then look at pictures of your grandparents when they were young. Fashions have changed even more since then! Haircuts, makeup, and clothing that may seem funny looking today were once considered to be the height of style and beauty.

Even the body shapes we think of as attractive have changed over the years. During the **Renaissance**, artists painted pictures of round-bellied, thick-legged women they considered to be beautiful. A few hundred years later,

What was the Renaissance? It was the period of European history between the 1300s and the 1600s.

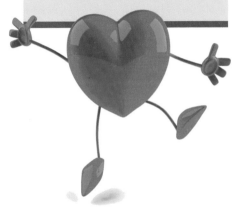

women wore something called a bustle under their dresses to make their hips and bottoms appear to be larger. In the 1890s, an actress named Lillian Russell was considered to be the "**ideal woman**"—and she weighed 200 pounds!

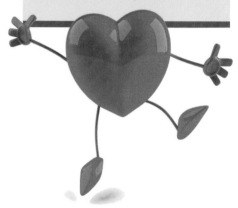

What does ideal mean? Something that's ideal is absolutely perfect. It measures up to the "perfect standard" we talked about in the last chapter.

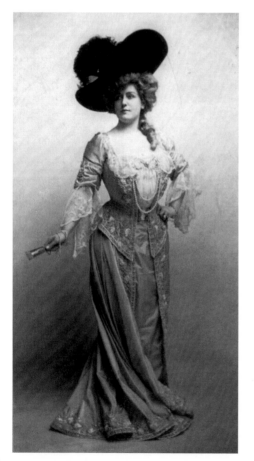

Appearance has to do with fashion—and fashions change all the time. Having fashionable clothes or a nice hairstyle are fine, but they don't really change who you are. A person wearing expensive clothes with her hair cut in the latest style could still be miserable on the inside. She could be sad or mean or sick.

Lillian Russell was an American actress and singer in the late 1800s. Despite being larger than the actresses of today, she was famous for her beauty and fashion.

But good health never goes out of style. And a person who is healthy is able to be the best he can be.

HEALTH AND BODY WEIGHT

People come in all different sizes and shapes. That's normal. Some people are tall and skinny, some are shorter and rounder. Some people have small bones, some people have large bones. Other people have lots of muscles. All these things will effect how much a person weighs. There's a wide range of weight that doctors consider to be healthy.

But people who are overweight or obese have more body fat than is healthy for their bodies. (Obesity is a more serious condition than being overweight is.) People who are overweight or obese can still be smart and pretty and funny, but the extra body fat they're carrying around can be dangerous. It puts them at risk for getting sick.

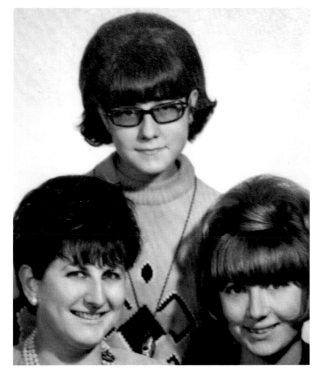

Look through some old family photos—you will most likely find some images that look funny to you because of the different hair and clothing styles.

Both children and adults who are overweight or obese are more likely to get diabetes. This is a disease where your body doesn't break down sugar the way it should. If you have diabetes, you will probably have to take medicine or have special shots every day to help your body process sugar normally. Diabetes can lead to other diseases as well, including blindness. It can make it hard for you to heal after a cut or injury.

Being overweight also increases your chances of having heart disease. This is an illness we usually connect with older people, but carrying too much weight around is hard on your heart, no matter how old you are. Even worse, the heavier you are, the harder it will probably be for you to run around and exercise. Your heart and lungs

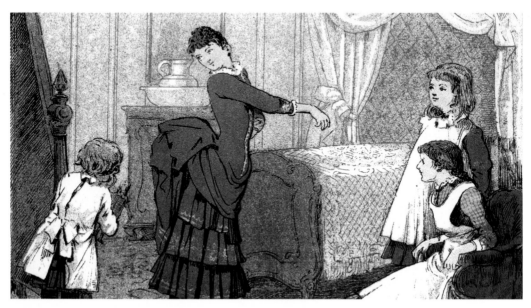

A bustle, shown here, was worn to make a woman's bottom and hips appear larger. This was because wider hips were thought to be very feminine and beautiful.

What is cancer?

Cancer is a disease that causes the cells in different parts of your body to grow too fast, to the point that they kill healthy cells.

What does high blood pressure and stroke mean?

High blood pressure is when blood pushes against the walls of the blood vessels harder than is normal. This tends to happen when the vessels become too narrow.

A stroke is when the cells in your brain suddenly die because they don't get enough blood.

What is your gallbladder?

Your gallbladder is an organ in your body that helps you digest fats.

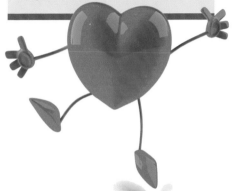

need exercise to be healthy. Today, more and more children are obese or overweight—and more and more children are getting heart disease.

Overweight children are also likely to stay that way as they grow up. Being obese or overweight when you are an adult can put you at risk for even more diseases. The extra weight puts strain on your joints, which can lead to arthritis, a disease that makes your joints swollen, stiff, and sore. Obesity may also cause certain kinds of **cancer**.

As people who are overweight or obese grow older, the added weight on their bodies can also lead to other problems, like **high blood pressure** (which increases your chances of having a **stroke**), **gallbladder** disease, and breathing problems. Being overweight can also mean that you have more problems handling your emotions. People who are obese or overweight are more likely to have **depression**.

HOW CAN YOU TELL IF YOU'RE OVERWEIGHT OR OBESE?

This question isn't as simple as you might think. It's not a question that can be answered by simply looking in the mirror, and it shouldn't be answered by comparing yourself to other kids your age either.

For one thing, some kids your age have begun going through **puberty**. Most kids gain weight more quickly during this time because the amounts of muscle, fat, and bone in their bodies change. But not everyone grows and develops on the same sched-

What is depression? Depression is an emotional illness that makes people feel very sad most of the time.

What's puberty? It's the stage in children's development when their bodies change to become like adults' bodies. During puberty, the body begins making hormones that spark physical changes like breast development in girls and larger testes in boys Both boys and girls will grow taller and heavier. Once these changes start, they continue for several years.

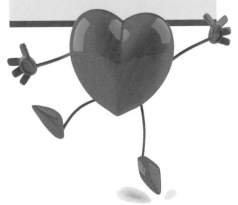

ule. This means that one healthy eleven-year-old might be small and skinny, while another might be nearly as tall and heavy as her mother. Some kids can start puberty when they're only eight years old, while others may wait until they're fourteen—and both are perfectly normal. Which is why it's also perfectly normal for two kids who are the same gender, height, and age to have very different weights.

Experts have figured out a way to help you know if you are in the healthy weight range for your height. It's called the body mass index or BMI. The BMI formula uses height and weight to come up with a BMI number. Though the formula is the same for adults and children, figuring out what the BMI number means is a little more complicated for kids. For kids, BMI is plotted on a growth chart that tells whether a child is underweight, healthy weight, overweight, or obese. Different BMI charts are used for boys and girls who are younger than twenty, because the amount of body fat differs between boys and girls. Also, the amount of body fat that is healthy is different, depending on whether you're a toddler or a teenager.

Each BMI chart is divided into percentiles. A child whose BMI is equal to or

> **DID YOU KNOW?**
>
> People who have eating disorders can be very, very thin—and still look in the mirror and think they are overweight!

greater than the 5th percentile and less than the 85th percentile is considered a healthy weight for his or her age. A child at or above the 85th percentile but less than the 95th percentile for age is considered overweight. A child at or above the 95th percentile is considered obese.

A child below the 5th percentile is considered underweight.

If you know how much you weigh and how tall you are, you can look at these charts and see for yourself whether you

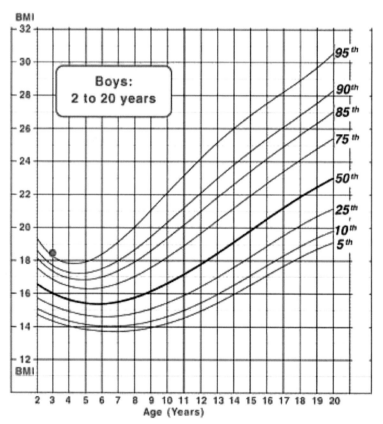

This BMI growth chart is used to find out if a boy between the ages of 2–20 is at a healthy weight for his height. The red dot shows that a three-year-old boy named Mike, who is 39.7 inches tall (100.8 cm) and weighs 41 pounds (18.6 kg), falls in the 95th percentile.

DID YOU KNOW?

The average person can expect to grow as much as 10 inches (25 centimeters) during puberty before reaching full adult height.

are overweight or obese—but it's also a good idea to talk to your doctor (even if that seems embarrassing). BMI is not always right, for some of the reasons we've already talked about, so a doctor will be better able to tell you if your weight is healthy or not.

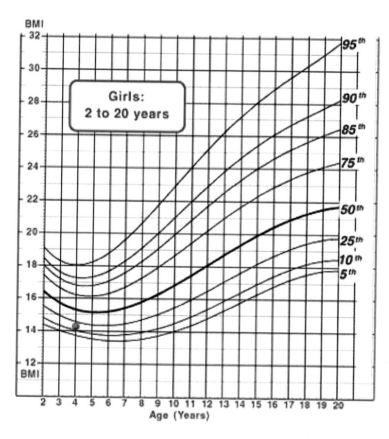

BMI

Girls:
2 to 20 years

95th
90th
85th
75th
50th
25th
10th
5th

Age (Years)

BMI-for-age charts are different for girls and boys. This one plots the BMI of a four-year-old girl named Mindy. She is 41.9 inches (106.4 cm) and 35.5 pounds (16.1 kg) and the red dot shows that she is in the 10th percentile.

WHAT'S THE ANSWER?

So if you're overweight, does that mean you should go on a diet?

No.

Studies have shown that BMI is not accurate for athletes. LeBron James is a fit, muscular basketball player, but because of his muscles his BMI is 27.5, which classifies him as overweight.

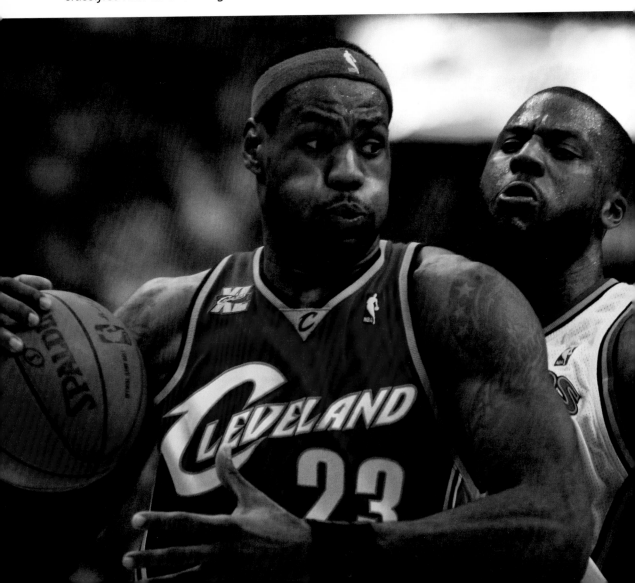

Experts say that dieting really isn't the best way to lose weight. People may lose weight on a diet, but after a while, most people start feeling frustrated—and HUNGRY! Sooner or later, they go back to eating the way they did before. Sometimes they eat even more than they did before.

The best way to be healthy is to change the way you live. The first step is to understand what your body really needs.

GOOD NUTRITION

All foods have calories, whether it's cookies or carrots, lettuce or ice cream, but some foods have more calories than others. This means that if you ate a pound of lettuce, you would have eaten only about 80 calories (and you would have had to eat about 16 cups of lettuce)—but if you ate a pound of chocolate chip cookies (about 10 cookies), you would have eaten 2,100 calories! That's a big difference.

Every day, your body needs **nutrition** from many kinds of foods. Different kinds of food contain different **nutrients**, and you need a balanced diet of all of them. That's why any diet plan that tells you to eat mostly one thing—or not at all of another thing—is probably not a very healthy way to eat. Your body needs carbohydrates, fats, protein, and minerals and vitamins every day. The only way to get what you need of these nutrients, is to eat lots of different kinds of healthy foods.

What does nutrition and nutrients mean? Nutrition is the process by which your body gets what it needs to live and grow from the food you eat. Nutrients are the things in food that help your body live and grow.

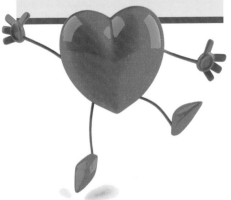

Eating a variety of foods is the best way to get the nutrition you need. Whole or unprocessed foods—foods that are as close as possible to the way they grew naturally, without being frozen, canned, or packaged—are the best choices for giving your body what it needs to stay healthy and grow properly.

Does this mean you have to give up foods like potato chips, candy bars, and cookies forever? No, it's okay to have these foods once in a while. Just don't eat too many of them. To choose healthier foods, check food labels, and then pick foods

GIRLS	Your age: Activity level:	9-13 years			14-18 years		
MyPyramid Food Group	Fill in YOUR Amounts	Inactive	Somewhat Active	Active	Inactive	Somewhat Active	Active
Fruits Group	cups	1½ cups	2 cups		1½ cups	2 cups	
Vegetables Group	cups	2 cups	2½ cups				3 cups
Milk Group	cups or equivalent	3 cups or equivalent					
Meat & Beans Group	ounces or equivalent	5 ounces or equivalent		5½ ounces or equivalent	5 ounces or equivalent	5½ ounces or equivalent	6½ ounces or equivalent
Grains Group	ounces or equivalent	5 ounces or equivalent	6 ounces or equivalent				8 ounces or equivalent

BOYS	Your age: Activity level:	9-13 years			14-18 years		
MyPyramid Food Group	Fill in YOUR Amounts	Inactive	Somewhat Active	Active	Inactive	Somewhat Active	Active
Fruits Group	cups	1½ cups	2 cups				2½ cups
Vegetables Group	cups	2½ cups		3 cups		3½ cups	4 cups
Milk Group	cups or equivalent	3 cups or equivalent					
Meat & Beans Group	ounces or equivalent	5 ounces or equivalent	5½ ounces or equivalent	6½ ounces or equivalent	6 ounces or equivalent	6½ ounces or equivalent	7 ounces or equivalent
Grains Group	ounces or equivalent	6 ounces or equivalent		8 ounces or equivalent	7 ounces or equivalent	9 ounces or equivalent	10 ounces or equivalent

Key	Less Food	Amounts for about 2,000 calories	More Food

WHERE DO YOU FIT?

Inactive Lifestyle.................. includes only the light physical activity of day-to-day life activities.

Somewhat Active Lifestyle... includes being physically active at a level equal to walking about 1½ to 3 miles at 3 to 4 miles per hour, beyond day-to-day life activities.

Active Lifestyle.................... includes being physically active at a level equal to walking more than 3 miles at 3 to 4 miles per hour, beyond day-to-day life activities.

Daily recommended amounts of each food group for girls and boys, ages 9–18.

that are high in vitamins and minerals. For example, if you're choosing a drink, a glass of milk is a good source of vitamin D, calcium, phosphorous, and potassium, but a glass of soda, has very few vitamins or minerals, if any—but it does have lots and lots of calories!

WHAT ELSE DO YOU NEED TO BE HEALTHY?

Good nutrition is an important part of good health, but your body also needs exercise in order to be the best it can be.

This doesn't mean you have to be an athlete, though! If you think sports are fun, then they're a great way to be sure your body gets the exercise it needs—but if you hate gym class, you can still find ways to exercise. Go for walks. Play with your dog. Find something active to do with a friend. Even helping your mom and dad with housework and yard work can be good exercise. It doesn't matter what you do, so long as you MOVE.

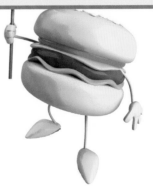

DID YOU KNOW?

Most children between the ages of 5 and 12 need between 1,200 and 2,000 calories a day. Exactly how much they need will depend on how active they are, whether they're in the midst of a growth spurt, and how big they are.

So be aware of how much television you're watching and how much time you're spending on the computer. As fun as these activities can be, they don't give you chances to move your body. Your body needs to exercise every day, so set aside some time when you turn off the television and computer—and do something that gets you moving. You'll be more apt to stick with it if it's something you think is fun.

The best way to be healthy, experts say, is to change your habits. Eat when you're hungry—but eat the foods your body needs. Find fun ways to get more exercise. Get plenty of sleep. Learn to take care of your body.

DID YOU KNOW?

Scientists have discovered the best combination of foods your body needs to be healthy. A diagram of this combination looks like a pyramid, with the foods you need to eat more at the bottom, and the foods you need to eat less at the top. The U.S. Department of Agriculture, the part of the American government that deals with food, farming, and nutrition, has created a picture called "MyPyramid" to help you understand better how much and what kinds of foods you need to eat in order to be healthy.

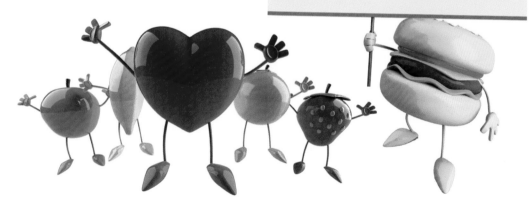

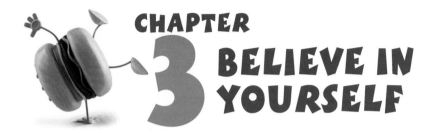

CHAPTER 3
BELIEVE IN YOURSELF

You'll feel more at home in your body if you believe in yourself. This means that no matter what you look like—whether you're chubby or skinny, tall or short—you know you're a person who has important things to give to the world. There's a part inside you that doesn't change, even if you're wearing your oldest and ugliest clothes or having the bad hair-day to end all hair-days.

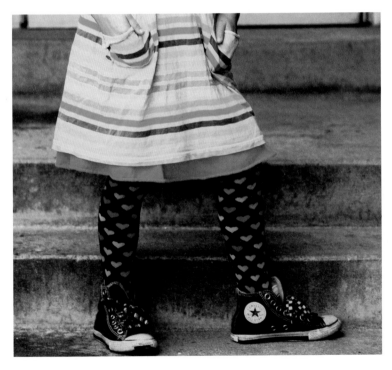

If you learn to love yourself, you are happy no matter what you look like on the outside!

MAKE THE MOST OF YOUR SOUL

Have you ever wondered why you were born? Have you ever thought about your purpose or the ultimate meaning of life? Have you ever imagined what happened to a loved one after she died? These kinds of questions move us to a deeper place than where our bodies live. Questions like these remind us that we are more than our bodies. We have a deeper self, what people sometimes call a soul.

Do you ever think about your soul? That deeper part of you might be clearest to you when you're lying awake thinking— or when you see something beautiful in nature, like a sunrise

What do you think about when you look up at the night sky?

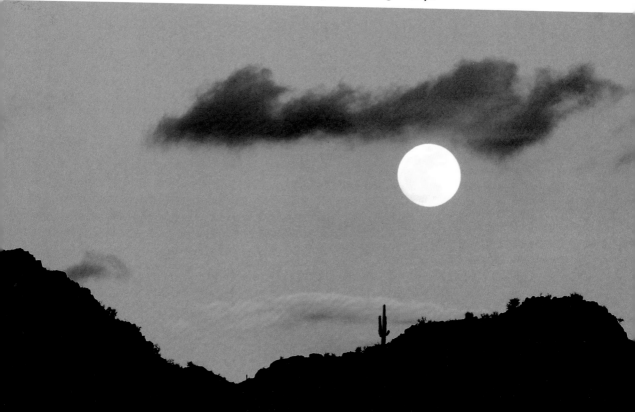

or a night sky full of stars—or when you're really happy or really sad.

Just as we need to take care of our bodies, we also need to care for our inner health. No matter what your religion (or even if you have no religion at all), certain things will help you feel more in touch with the deep, inner you.

QUIET THOUGHT

Take time to think. Ask big questions about God, the universe, and what life means. Even if you don't know the answers, just

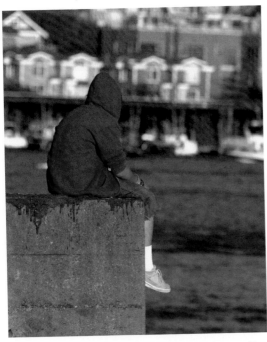

asking the questions is good for your soul. Think about what's *really* important to you—or what you'd like to do when you grow up—or how you'd like to change the world. If you believe in a Supreme Being, talk to him (or her). Some people call these times prayer or meditation. Times like this can help you feel calm and peaceful. They help your soul feel more at home in your body.

It is healthy to spend time with yourself just thinking, praying, or meditating. These moments help you know yourself better, and can make you happier with the way to look and feel.

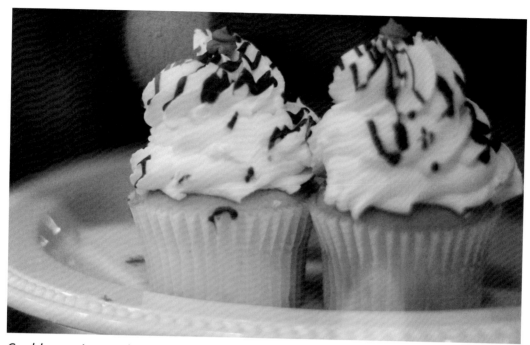

Could you give up dessert for a week? Or video games? Fasting from something you love can help you find other things to do or think about.

FASTS

A fast is a period of time when you choose to do without something. It doesn't mean you've given it up forever. It just means you're taking a break from it to make room for something else to grow.

Have you ever thought about taking a break from television for a whole week? That would be a television fast. Or how about not eating any dessert for a day? That would be a dessert fast. If you chose to give up texting for twenty-four hours, that would be a telephone fast. Or you could go on a computer fast.

The point of a fast is to change something about your day-to-day lifestyle so you can focus more on the deeper issues of life. It gives you a chance to think about other things. It lets your soul have room to grow.

RETREAT

A retreat is a time to get away from your normal life. It could be a family vacation—or it could be something as short and simple as going for a walk by yourself. Retreats are times when we shut ourselves away from things like homework and chores, the television and the computer, cell phones and even our friends, so that we can focus on our inner life. Afterwards, we usually find we can cope better with the stress in our lives. We see things more clearly.

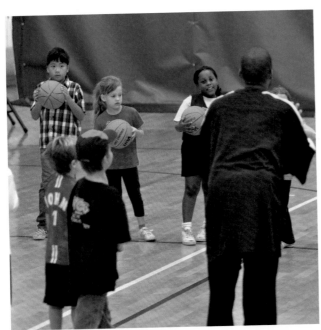

Remember, you won't be the best at everything, and that is ok! Maybe you have trouble in gym class, but are a talented artist—learn to recognize the things you are good at to build your self-confidence.

Sometimes people combine retreats, fasts, and times of quiet thought. It doesn't really matter how you make time for your inner life, so long as you do. No matter what your body size, type, color, shape, or appearance, your soul is important. The more in touch you are with the "inner you," the more comfortable you're likely to be with the "outer you."

Sometimes people combine retreats, fasts, and times of quiet thought. It doesn't really matter how you make time for your inner life, so long as you do. No matter what your body size, type, color, shape, or appearance, your soul is important. The more in touch you are with the "inner you," the more comfortable you're likely to be with the "outer you."

BUILDING YOUR SELF-CONFIDENCE

Even when you take time for the inner you, you still have to live in the outer world! Out there, believing in yourself isn't always easy.

All of us sometimes worry that we don't measure up to those around us. If you have problems believing in yourself, try these things to boost your confidence level:

1. Don't expect yourself to be perfect. Being good at something doesn't mean you have to be perfect at it. Remember that everyone has both good points

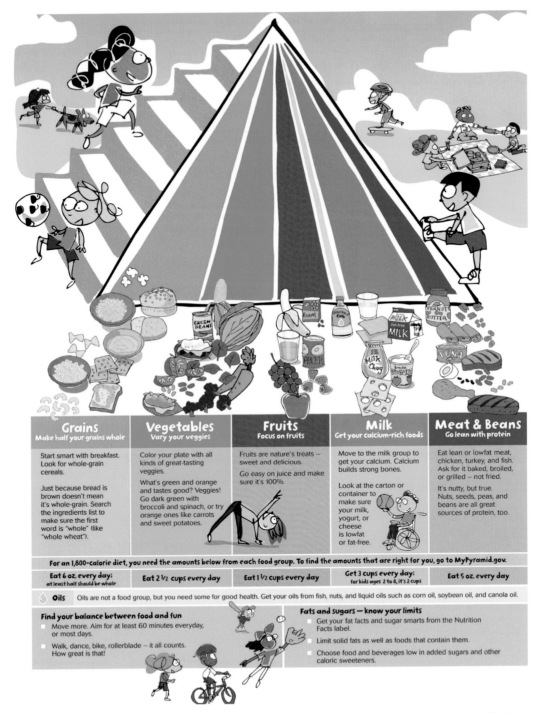

Grains
Make half your grains whole

Start smart with breakfast. Look for whole-grain cereals.

Just because bread is brown doesn't mean it's whole-grain. Search the ingredients list to make sure the first word is "whole" (like "whole wheat").

Vegetables
Vary your veggies

Color your plate with all kinds of great-tasting veggies.

What's green and orange and tastes good? Veggies! Go dark green with broccoli and spinach, or try orange ones like carrots and sweet potatoes.

Fruits
Focus on fruits

Fruits are nature's treats — sweet and delicious.

Go easy on juice and make sure it's 100%.

Milk
Get your calcium-rich foods

Move to the milk group to get your calcium. Calcium builds strong bones.

Look at the carton or container to make sure your milk, yogurt, or cheese is lowfat or fat-free.

Meat & Beans
Go lean with protein

Eat lean or lowfat meat, chicken, turkey, and fish. Ask for it baked, broiled, or grilled — not fried.

It's nutty, but true. Nuts, seeds, peas, and beans are all great sources of protein, too.

For an 1,800-calorie diet, you need the amounts below from each food group. To find the amounts that are right for you, go to MyPyramid.gov.

Eat 6 oz. every day: at least half should be whole	Eat 2½ cups every day	Eat 1½ cups every day	Get 3 cups every day: for kids ages 2 to 8, it's 2 cups	Eat 5 oz. every day

Oils   Oils are not a food group, but you need some for good health. Get your oils from fish, nuts, and liquid oils such as corn oil, soybean oil, and canola oil.

Find your balance between food and fun

- Move more. Aim for at least 60 minutes everyday, or most days.
- Walk, dance, bike, rollerblade — it all counts. How great is that!

Fats and sugars — know your limits

- Get your fat facts and sugar smarts from the Nutrition Facts label.
- Limit solid fats as well as foods that contain them.
- Choose food and beverages low in added sugars and other caloric sweeteners.

Learning to lead a healthier lifestyle can be a part of learning to like yourself. The food pyramid gives advice for healthy eating and activity.

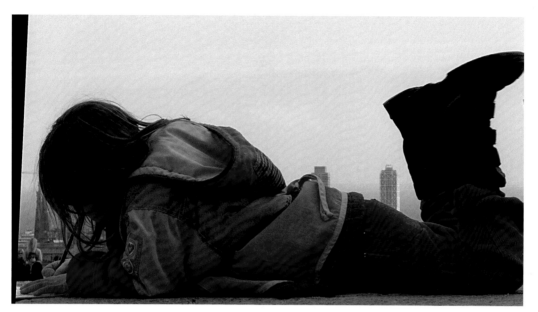

Write a list of things you do really well. Read it as a pick-me-up when you are feeling down.

and bad, but no one—including you—is really all bad or a complete screw-up. We all have things we do well and things we don't do as well as others.

2. Turn off the voice inside your head that is always putting you down. Most of us have a little voice like that— but those voices are liars! Learn not to listen. Every time you're tempted to tell yourself how fat, ugly, or stupid you are, pretend that those thoughts are part of a message on TV commercial. Imagine turning using a remote control to switch the channel every time one of those thoughts pops into your head.

3. Make a list of things people you respect (friends, parents, coaches, teachers) say you do well or like about you. Keep that list where you can read it every time you begin to doubt yourself.

4. Write down anything you do well. Maybe you know how to be a good friend. Maybe you can help others calm down when they're upset. Maybe you can smile even when life gets you down. Maybe you can bake great cookies or write nice e-mails. Maybe you're a good student, a talented musician, or someone who can draw cartoons really well. Whatever it is, write it down— and then read over your list often. Focus on what you CAN do rather than what you CAN'T.

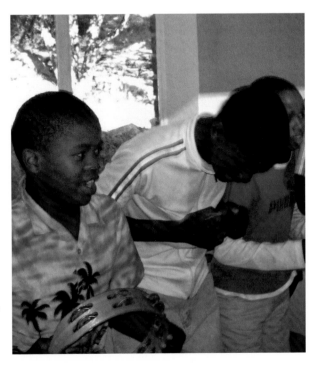

You are unique—enjoy your talents and don't worry about how you compare to your friends or siblings.

5. Stop comparing yourself to other people. You are not going to have the same strengths someone else has—but you have your own! You are unique, one-of-a-kind. That means you have something to offer this world that is all your own. No one sees things quite the same way you do. Only you can offer your opinion or ideas on things.

6. Don't get angry with yourself or feel sad if you make mistakes. Everyone makes mistakes. We all have weaknesses. They are nothing to be ashamed of. They're just part of being human. Our strengths and weaknesses are part of what make us who we are. They are what make us need each other. What a boring world we'd live in if everyone was perfect!

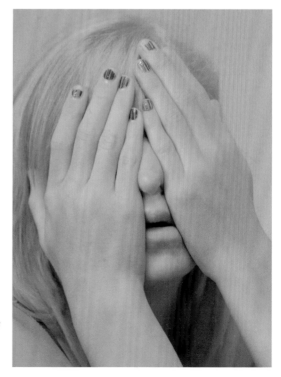

Don't get mad or upset at yourself about mistakes—they happen to everyone!

7. Look at your failures and embarrassments as chances for you to grow and change. Learn to laugh at yourself. Remember, everyone has moments like these. We can learn from these things and become better for them.

8. Make a list of your interests. What do you like doing? What interests you? If you could do anything or be anyone, what would it be? Your interests and dreams are part of what make you YOU.

9. Do something new. Volunteer to help others. Try a new sport. Write a letter to your local paper. Make a new friend. Step outside your comfort zone. Stretch your boundaries.

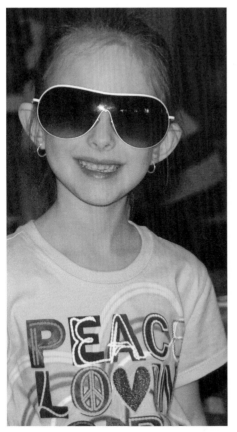

10. Take care of yourself, mind, body, and soul. Get enough sleep. Exercise regularly. Eat right. Take time to laugh. Spend time with the people who make you feel good about yourself. Make time to dream.

Be proud of your differences—they make you special.

You have the power to make the world a better place. Use your power!

FREE TO BE YOU

Everybody in this world has an imperfect body. We all have things about our bodies we'd like to hide. But there are more important things in life than what we look like, things like our health, as well as love, friendship, kindness.

People need to feel like they belong. They need to feel loved. They need to feel as though they have something important to do in the world. And none of those things depend on appearance. It doesn't matter whether you are fat or skinny, ugly or beautiful. The important things are found deep inside.

Being at home in your own body lets you start to become the best YOU you can be. It gives you the **confidence** to take care of yourself and be healthy. And it gives you the strength and courage to reach out to others.

What does confidence mean? It means freedom from doubt. It means you believe in yourself and your abilities.

There's only one of you. So make a difference in the world that only you can make. And enjoy yourself!

READ MORE ABOUT IT

Beck, Debra. *My Feet Aren't Ugly! A Girl's Guide to Loving Herself from the Inside Out.* New York: Beaufort, 2007.

Bowen, Connie. *I Believe in Me*. Unity Village, Mo.: Unity Books, 2007.

Gay, Kathlyn. *Am I Fat?* Berkeley Heights, N.J.: Enslow, 2006.

Jimerson, M. N. *Childhood Obesity.* Farmington Hills, Mich.: Lucent, 2008.

Johnson, Susan and Laurel Mellin. *Just for Kids! (Obesity Prevention Workbook).* San Anselmo, Calif.: Balboa Publishing, 2002.

Mysko, Claire. *You're Amazing! A No-Pressure Guide to Being Your Best Self.* Cincinatti, Ohio: Adams Media, 2008.

Prim-Ed. *Lifestyle Choices*. Boston: Prim-Ed, 2005.

Wann, Marilyn. *Fat! So? Because You Don't Have to Apologize for Your Size.* Berkeley. Calif.: Ten Speed Press, 2009.

Wilde, Jerry. *Hot Stuff to Help Kids Cheer Up: The Depression and Self-Esteem Workbook*. Naperville, Ill.: Sourcebooks Jabberwocky, 2007.

FIND OUT MORE ON THE INTERNET

About Our Kids: Obesity and Overweight
www.aboutourkids.org/aboutour/articles/gr_obesity_03.html

American Obesity Association
www.obesity.org

Definition and Classification of Obesity
www.endotext.org/obesity/obesity1/obesityframe1.htm

Empowered Kids
www.treatingeatingdisorders.com/empoweredkidz/

Environmental Contributions to Obesity
www.endotext.org/obesity/obesity7/obesity7.htm

The Food Guide Pyramid
kidshealth.org/kid/stay_healthy/food/pyramid.html

Food and Nutrition Information Center
www.nal.usda.gov/fnic

Healthy Food Choices: Nutrition Explorations
www.nutritionexplorations.org/parents/health-food.asp

The Learning Center
www.hebs.scot.nhs.uk/learningcentre/obesity/intro/index.cfm

MyPyramid for Kids
www.mypyramid.gov/Kids/

Statistics Related to Overweight and Obesity
win.niddk.nih.gov/statistics/index.htm

The websites listed on this page were active at the time of publication. The publisher is not responsible for websites that have changed their address or discontinued operation since the date of publication. The publisher will review and update the websites upon each reprint.

INDEX

PICTURE CREDITS

ABOUT THE AUTHOR

Rae Simons has ghostwritten several adult books on dieting and obesity. She is also the author of more than thirty young adult books. She lives in upstate New York, where she tries hard to get enough exercise and eat healthy foods.